INFERTILITY
AND MEDICALLY ASSISTED CONCEPTION

by
Agneta Sutton

*All booklets are published thanks to the
generous support of the members of the
Catholic Truth Society*

CATHOLIC TRUTH SOCIETY
PUBLISHERS TO THE HOLY SEE

2

CONTENTS

The Author

Agneta Sutton is an Associate Lecturer in Christian
Ethics at University College Chichester, with a Ph.D in
theology from King's College London. She has
published widely in the field of medical ethics, in
particular in the area of reproductive medicine and
genetics. She has a regular column in the Catholic Times
and is Associate Editor of Ethics and Medicine. She is
married and has 4 adult children.

THE LINACRE CENTRE

The Linacre Centre is the only Catholic institution of its kind specialising in the field of healthcare ethics in Great Britain and Ireland. As such it provides a unique service to the Catholic community in these islands and more particularly to Catholics working in the field of healthcare. The Centre also exists to assist the teaching authorities within the Church in addressing bioethical issues, and to communicate and defend the Church's moral teaching in debates over public policy and legislation in the United Kingdom.

The Centre has built up a large bioethics library at the Hospital of St John and St Elizabeth in London. It has three fulltime research fellows who are able to give time and thought to new and difficult issues in bioethics and it is also able to call upon the help of a range of experts in medicine, law, philosophy, theology and history. The Centre is affiliated to the Ave Maria School of Law, Ann Arbor, Michigan. It publishes reports, organises conferences and lectures, and does consultancy work for individuals and for other organisations. The co-operation of the Linacre Centre in publishing the *CTS Explanations* series of booklets is intended to advance this work of providing clear Catholic teaching on bioethical issues.

INTRODUCTION

The first IVF or 'test-tube' baby, Louise Brown, was born in 1978. Her birth marked a new era in reproductive medicine. Today IVF is a rather commonplace procedure. The ethics of the technology is no longer a matter of public debate, except when the issue of designer babies is raised or when stored embryos are the objects of parental disputes. However, it is not only designer babies and stored embryos that raise ethical questions in connection with IVF and many other reproductive technologies. These issues simply highlight one of the fundamental moral concerns in relation to the new technologies, namely the commodification of human life. That is, the child is treated as a product and possession. Reproductive technologies that replace, rather than restore or assist, the sexual act depersonalise the child as well as the very process of conception. New life becomes the product of a technological process. This is especially obvious when the embryo comes into being outside the human body. Then the process of conception becomes the result of laboratory procedures, the mere coupling of gametes in a dish away from the warmth of the human embrace and the protective environment of the maternal body. Accessible in the petri-dish, the embryo becomes subjected to quality control and selection, just like artefacts in general. Thousands of embryos have been wasted and discarded following IVF.

This kind of wastage and depersonalisation of human life in the context of medically assisted conception has a bearing on the way we see ourselves and our children. It affects our understanding of what it means to be human. This is why it is important to know that there are alternatives to technologies that replace, rather than restore or assist, normal sexual conception. Reproductive technologies that replace the sexual act may be presented as ordinary medical care to those who seek fertility treatment. But, as is shown in this booklet, they entail a failure to appreciate and respect the personal dimension of the human subject.

The aim of this booklet is to explain the different options of assisted conception and their moral and anthropological implications. The first chapter opens with an explanation of the woman's reproductive cycle and the main causes of infertility. Then an account is provided of how infertile couples may be helped in order to restore - if only temporarily - their ability to conceive by means of natural intercourse. This section is followed by descriptions of technologies that neither restore nor assist sexual conception but rather replace it. In other words, a distinction is made between treatment that enables couples to conceive by means of human intercourse and treatment that circumvents the problem by means of technology.

The status of the human embryo is discussed in the second chapter. The first part of the chapter explains and dismisses a number of philosophical objections to the view that the newly conceived embryo is an individual human being, a member of the human family. The second part presents the Church's teaching on respect for the human embryo.

The Church's teaching on respect for procreation is explained in the third chapter. The focus is on *Donum Vitae*, a document published by the Congregation for the Doctrine of the Faith in 1987 and also on John Paul II's Apostolic Exhortation of 1981, *Familiaris Consortio*, and his *Letter to Families* of 1994. It is explained why the child should be the fruit of married love and why techniques of assisted reproduction that do not allow couples to conceive by means of intercourse depersonalise the couple and their child and so fail to respect human dignity.

INFERTILITY: ITS CAUSES AND TREATMENT

The reproductive period in the life of men and women

The reproductive time of life for men as well as for women begins with puberty. However, the number of their fertile years differs. The reproductive time of life ends in the case of women with menopause, whereas men may remain fertile throughout life even if their fertility declines with age. Moreover, the fertility of women is cyclical, whereas that of men is not. While women are fertile only a few days each month, men are equally fertile every day of the month.

Throughout the reproductive years of a woman's life a mature ovum (egg) is released each month from her ovaries. This is called ovulation and it takes place midway between two menstrual periods or, more precisely, some 14 days before the next expected period. At ovulation the ovum is picked up by the fallopian tube. It is in the fallopian tube that fertilisation normally takes place. If the ovum is not fertilised within 12-24 hours of ovulation it perishes and a new period follows 12-14 days later. However, because the sperm survives longer than the ovum, intercourse up to four or five days before ovulation can result in fertilisation, as can intercourse one day after. Hence, in actual fact, the fertile days of the woman's cycle number about five or six. The woman is, however, most likely to conceive around the time of ovulation.

If the ovum is fertilised the resulting embryo travels down the fallopian tube to the uterus (womb). This takes about 3-4 days. Having arrived in the uterus the embryo will begin implanting itself in the uterine wall.

Infertility

Most couples who wish to have a child and who have regular intercourse will conceive within half a year. But this does not mean that a couple is infertile if they take longer to conceive. Usually a couple is not described as infertile unless they have been trying (unsuccessfully) to have a child for at least two years. About one in six couples are infertile in the sense of experiencing difficulty in conceiving.

One may distinguish between primary and secondary infertility. The former term refers to patients who have never conceived; the latter to patients who have previously conceived but have subsequently found themselves unable to do so. Either type of infertility may be brought about by a number of causes.

In the case of men the most common cause of infertility - or subfertility - is poor sperm quality.

For women the most common causes of impaired fertility are the ones listed as follows:

1) Blocked or defective fallopian tubes. In this situation the ovum may be prevented from entering the tube, or the passage through the tube of either ovum or sperm may be obstructed. This is a very common cause of infertility, not least in the case of secondary infertility. About 33% of cases of infertility are caused by faulty fallopian tubes (Human Fertilisation and Embryology Authority (HFEA), *Patient's Guide to Infertility and IVF*, 2001). Surgery to repair the fallopian tubes might be successful. However, most patients today are recommended to avail themselves of IVF.

Often the cause of blocked tubes is an infection. Women with several sexual partners are more prone to infections than women who stay with one partner only. This is because of the risk of contracting sexually transmitted diseases. The IUD (intra-uterine device) may also cause infection. Another cause of infection is procured abortion.

2) Endometriosis (misplaced uterine lining) is another relatively common cause of infertility in women, especially primary infertility. It is the cause of female infertility in some 8% of cases (HFEA, *op.cit.*).

3) Immunological factors. The woman may have developed anti-sperm antibodies preventing her from conceiving together with her partner. Anti-sperm

antibodies may also be found in a man's own semen. Hormone treatment helps in some cases.

4) Unexplained infertility. This is the most common situation and accounts for about 42% of cases.

It is important to realise that many couples who think that they are infertile will find that they spontaneously conceive even if they seek no medical assistance. Often the mere stress of trying to have a baby renders the woman temporarily infertile.

Different forms of treatment

Treatment restoring function and allowing conception by means of intercourse

In many cases infertility may be overcome by means of drugs or surgery in a way that restores reproductive function and allows conception by means of intercourse. These kinds of treatment do not depersonalise conception. They do not make it a purely medical or technical undertaking. For in this situation conception involves not merely the coupling of gametes to form an embryo. The human embryo is conceived in the act of love between a man and a woman. It is the crowning and fulfilment of their mutual self-giving in their loving embrace. Why this is important for our understanding of ourselves as human beings will be explained in Chapter 3.

There are number of treatments which fall in this category.

1) Hormone treatment may overcome infertility in women who do not ovulate regularly, thus enabling them to conceive by normal intercourse.

2) Surgery may correct blocked or defective fallopian tubes, allowing the ovum to be fertilised by intercourse. Surgery may also be used to correct other structural defects in the female reproductive tract.

3) Immunological problems are sometimes resolved by means of hormone treatment. If successful, this treatment too will allow conception by means of intercourse.

4) Endometriosis is sometimes successfully treated by surgery, allowing the woman to become pregnant as a result of intercourse.

Naprotechnology

It is important for Catholic couples to realise that the Church does not object to the use of technology as such. It does not object to tubal surgery to restore tubal function. Nor is it opposed to the careful use of hormones to restore fertility. Furthermore, the Church does not object to other procedures that make intercourse more effective, such as using an instrument to move sperm deposited in the woman's vagina further up the woman's reproductive tract in order to achieve conception. The Church is only opposed to techniques that by-pass normal intercourse and/or use donated gametes (sperm or ova).

For example, the Pope Paul VI Institute for the Study of Human Reproduction in the United States has developed a programme that involves teaching couples how to track the woman's cycle and observe physical changes in her body in order to understand her fertility and know when in the month she is most likely to conceive. Working together with the couple, doctors provide medical care that is based on standardised and objective monitoring of normal and naturally occurring biological signs in the female body. These signs give the clue to what treatment, if any, may be required. Any treatment provided is supportive of the natural cycle.

The naprotechnology system monitors the reproductive function of the woman and can be used to assess what form of hormone treatment she may need or to identify ovarian cysts as well as the effects of stress. It may also be used to assess chronic discharges and unusual bleeding, whether to promote natural conception or to protect the woman's health as a whole.

Treatments that by-pass sexual intercourse

When people speak of the new reproductive technologies they usually have in mind technologies that by-pass the sexual act. There are a number of such techniques. Several of them are regulated by the HFEA. Treatments that belong to this category can only be given in clinics that have been granted a licence by the HFEA. The procedures in question include all forms of treatment involving gamete donation (egg or sperm donation) as well as IVF and related procedures. The HFEA also regulates embryo research and the storage of gametes and embryos. (The HFEA is the source of the statistics concerning success rates and risks cited in this chapter.)

The methods of medically assisted conception by-passing sexual intercourse are listed below.

1) Artificial insemination by husband (AIH)

2) Donor Insemination (DI)

3) *In vitro* fertilisation (IVF) (and related procedures)

4) Gamete intra-fallopian transfer (GIFT) and zygote intra-fallopian transfer (ZIFT)

AIH
Artificial insemination by husband

Why do some couples use AIH?

AIH may be offered to couples in the case of low sperm count (that is, if the man is failing to produce sufficient sperm in normal intercourse) or if the quality of the sperm is poor. It may also be offered if the woman's cervical mucus contains anti-sperm antibodies or is otherwise abnormal or absent, thus preventing the passage of sperm from the vagina to the uterus. It may likewise be used in the case of cervical structural problems blocking the passage of sperm from the vagina to the uterus.

What is involved in AIH?

The man's semen is deposited in the woman's uterus by means of a syringe. The semen is usually obtained by masturbation.

What are the risks and success rates?

The medical risks are small. The pregnancy rate varies, depending on the problem. Whether the procedure results in pregnancy and birth depends very much on the nature of the problem. In the case of low sperm count or poor quality sperm, as well as in the case of anti-sperm antibodies, IVF is usually the preferred option.

DI
Donor Insemination

Why do people use DI?

Donor Insemination may be offered in the case of male infertility due to low sperm count or poor quality sperm. The number of couples resorting to DI has decreased apace with the increased use of IVF to overcome male infertility, suggesting that most couples prefer to have a child who is genetically completely theirs.

DI may also be offered if the husband risks passing on a medical condition to the next generation if he fathers any children. In addition it may be used to allow lesbian couples or single women to have children. This is despite the fact that the Human Fertilisation and Embryology Act 1990 specifically mentions that the child's need for a father must be taken into account before a decision is taken about medically assisted conception involving sperm donation.

What is involved?

The insemination procedure is the same as in the case of AIH. Sperm donors are aged between 18 and 55. They are screened for a number of diseases, including AIDS, syphilis and hepatitis B. They are also screened to make sure that they are not carriers of a gene for cystic fibrosis, the most common genetic disease among people of European origin. The semen is normally stored for a minimum period of six months before it is used. This is to allow the donor to be re-tested for disease before his semen is used. Sometimes anti-bodies to, for example, AIDS do not show up on the first test. The donor's blood group will be determined, and his general health and medical records will be examined. In order to match donor and recipients, a number of physical characteristics of the donor, such as skin colour, eye colour, blood group, hair colour and body build will also be recorded. At present no personal identification of the donor is provided to the person or couple wanting a child, or to the offspring him/herself. However, the anonymity of donors is now subject to debate and the situation may change in the future.

In the case of a married couple being treated by sperm donation, the husband is registered as the father of the child on the latter's birth certificate, provided he has agreed to the arrangement. If he has not agreed to the arrangement, the child is registered as fatherless. Those who argue that the child conceived by donation ought to be allowed to find out who his or her father is point out that the present situation promotes deception. Proof of this is to be found in the fact that only a small minority of couples using sperm donation tell the child about his or her true origin.

What are the risks and success rates?

Even with careful screening of donors, the woman is exposed to a certain risk of infection. In the case of donor insemination with the help of a male friend and a DI kit, the risk of infection is increased, since the donor would not have been screened. There is also a small but non-negligible risk that the donor will pass on a hereditary condition.

According to the HFEA's current Patient's Guide to DI, women under 30 achieve a live birth rate of 10-12% per treatment cycle, but the success rate decreases in older women. Women aged 35-39 have a 9% chance of a live birth per treatment cycle, while women over 40 have only a 3-4% chance of a successful pregnancy.

Are donors paid?

Donors are paid £15 per donation plus expenses. It may be commented that the very fact that the donor is paid shows that the child itself, as well as the donor's sperm, is being treated as a commodity.

IVF
In-Vitro Fertilisation

IVF is short for *in vitro* fertilisation, which means fertilisation in a glass dish (though the dish may, in fact, be made of plastic). The important point is that fertilisation takes place outside the body. (IVF is another procedure that is regulated by the HFEA.)

Under what circumstances may a couple be offered IVF?

A couple might be offered IVF when the woman has damaged or blocked fallopian tubes, or endometriosis, or when the man has a low sperm count or reduced sperm quality, as well as in cases of unexplained infertility. IVF may also be used to overcome immune problems or when sperm are prevented from entering the uterus because of a defective structure of the cervix. A special IVF technique, ICSI (Intra-cytoplasmic sperm injection) may be offered to overcome male infertility.

While IVF is usually offered as a form of treatment helping a couple to have a child who is genetically their own, it may also involve gamete donation. For example, older women may avail themselves of ovum donation in connection with IVF, as this increases their chances of having a baby. Some couples may use donated sperm if the man is infertile. Others may avail themselves of either egg or sperm donation in order to avoid passing on a genetic condition.

What is involved?

IVF is a complicated and burdensome procedure, involving a number of separate steps.

1) Stimulation of the ovaries to promote super-ovulation

Different hormonal drug regimes may be used first to suppress the body's own hormone regulation and then to stimulate the ovaries to over-produce, that is, to produce not one ripe ovum as in the normal case but a multitude of ripe ova. The reason for seeking to produce several ripe ova in one and the same cycle is that it is thought that the chances of achieving a pregnancy are increased if more than one embryo is placed in the uterus.

However, according to new HFEA regulations, no more than two embryos may be placed in the uterus, except in very special circumstances when a maximum of three may be inserted at the same time. The grounds for lowering the number of embryos that may normally be placed in the uterus - from three to two - are the risks attached to a multiple pregnancy, such as premature delivery and low birth weight. Small and premature babies are exposed to more medical complications.

It should also be pointed out that ovarian stimulation is not without risks and discomfort. Not only may the woman have to have daily injections for an extended period of a month or so but, in addition, she may suffer various unpleasant and even dangerous side-effects.

2) Egg collection

When the ova (eggs) have ripened, they are collected. This may be done by passing an ultrasound probe into the vagina to visualise the ovaries, thereby allowing a needle to be guided through the top of the vagina to suck up the ova. The woman would be sedated for the procedure to reduce her discomfort. In some cases the egg collection may be performed passing through the abdominal wall under ultrasound guidance. In this situation a local anaesthetic would normally be used, though some women may prefer a general anaesthetic.

Ultrasound-guided egg collection may take between 20 and 40 minutes in which time about a dozen eggs or more may be collected. Afterwards the woman has to rest for a couple of hours before she can go home.

3) Sperm collection

The man's sperm is usually obtained by masturbation. This has to be done in the morning the same day as egg collection takes place.

4) Fertilisation

After egg collection the ova are usually incubated for a short time before sperm are added separately to each ovum. Usually several embryos will result from this process.

5) Embryo transfer

Two or three days after egg collection two (or very rarely three) embryos may be transferred to the uterus. In some cases embryos are transferred some six days after egg collection at the blastocyst stage. In either case, the transfer only takes place after the embryos have been examined under a microscope and 'high quality' ones have been selected. Usually this means there are a number of embryos left over: so-called 'spare' embryos. 'Spare' embryos thought to be of 'high quality' may be frozen and stored for future use by the couple. Alternatively, they may be donated to other couples. Other embryos may be used in embryo research, while many are immediately destroyed. Each option requires the couple's consent. The fact that many embryos are destroyed in connection with IVF is one of the main moral objections to the procedure.

The actual placement of the embryos requires no anaesthetic. A fine plastic tube containing the embryos is passed through the vagina into the uterus where the embryos are injected. A pregnancy test is performed some 14 days later. If it is positive an ultrasound scan is performed after another couple of weeks to make sure that the woman is pregnant.

Risks and success rates

As noted, IVF exposes the child to special medical risks, mainly because it is associated with multiple pregnancy and low birth weight.

The main medical risks to the mother are those attached to ovarian stimulation. However, the extraction of the ova is an invasive procedure and as such it involves a certain risk. In addition, there are risks linked to the psychological well-being of the woman and, indeed, her husband. IVF is time-consuming and burdensome. It involves a certain amount of anxiety. There is anxiety about the very procedures themselves and a fear of failure. Should the fear of failure be realised, there is the agony of disappointment coupled with the question of whether to try again or give up.

According to HFEA statistics released in August 2002, in the UK the overall chance of bringing home a live baby after IVF is 25.1% per cycle started, in women aged less than 38, compared with 21.8% for all ages. In cycles in which egg collection has successfully taken place the live birth rate is higher: 26.8% in women below 38, and 23.5% counting women of all age groups. The live birth rate rises further if not only egg collection but also embryo transfer has successfully taken place. In this situation it is 28.8% in women below 38 and, and overall for women of all ages 24.3%. These results may sound very reassuring. However, they mean that in more than 70% of cases in which an embryo is transferred to the uterus, the woman goes home empty handed; that is, without a baby. This in itself is an indication of the trauma suffered by thousands of women and couples.

ICSI

Intra-cytoplasmic sperm injection (ICSI) is a special IVF technique in which a single sperm is injected directly into the centre of an ovum. This is done under a microscope using a very fine needle. ICSI is used to overcome male infertility due to poor quality sperm or low sperm count. It is also used when there has been poor fertilisation of ova during conventional IVF treatment mixing sperm and ova. The sperm is obtained by masturbation or directly from the testis under general anaesthesia, and the 'best quality' sperm is selected.

The live birth rate is much the same as in the case of conventional IVF, but couples seeking ICSI are warned that offspring of men with a low sperm count are at increased risk of inheriting genetic anomalies and infertility. There are also certain risks attached to the piercing of the outer and inner membranes of the ovum; it is possible that the development of the embryo could be disturbed. According to information available on the website of The Assisted Conception Unit, University College, London, 'minor abnormalities occur in up to 20% of ICSI babies, compared with 15% of the population'.

In short, IVF entails a number of risks to women and children. The woman's natural cycle is totally suppressed so that her ovaries may be artificially stimulated to produce a multitude of ova, for the production of a multitude of embryos, most of whom will become 'spare' embryos and be left to die or to face an uncertain future in storage. IVF often results in multiple pregnancy with the attendant risks to the health of the babies produced. It exposes men, women and children to medical technology that commodifies human life by treating the embryo as a disposable product and the couple as providers of raw material for its manufacture.

GIFT
Gamete intra-fallopian transfer

Under what circumstances may GIFT be offered?

GIFT is short for gamete intra-fallopian transfer. The procedure may be used provided the woman has at least one functioning fallopian tube. It may be offered when the cause of infertility is unknown, when the woman has endometriosis, when her cervical mucus contains anti-sperm antibodies and in cases of male infertility. It may also be used with donated sperm when DI has failed. It falls under the regulatory authority of the HFEA only if donated gametes are used.

What is involved?

In GIFT sperm and ova are deposited together directly in the fallopian tube for fertilisation to take place there. Like IVF, GIFT involves ovarian stimulation to produce several ripe ova in the same cycle. The ova are retrieved as in IVF or by means of laparoscopy under general anaesthesia. If laparoscopy is used, the procedure may be undertaken on the same occasion as the gametes are deposited in the fallopian tube, since that too will involve laparoscopy. Semen is collected as in IVF, put in a centrifuge and washed and then placed in a test tube. 'Active' sperm that swim to the surface of the tube are then placed in a thin catheter. Two mature ova may be placed in the same or another catheter to be transported with the sperm to the fallopian tube.

Risks and success rates

The risks for the woman are essentially the same as in IVF with the added risk attached to the general anaesthesia accompanying the laparoscopy procedure. The success rate of GIFT is similar to that of IVF.

ZIFT

ZIFT, short for zygote intra-fallopian transfer, may be described as a variation of both IVF and GIFT. The difference between GIFT and ZIFT is that in ZIFT newly conceived one-cell embryos (zygotes), rather than gametes, are transferred to the fallopian tube. This means that ova are fertilised in a dish as in IVF, but the resulting embryos are not 'cultured' and so not allowed to start cell division as they would in the case of ordinary IVF.

RESPECT FOR THE HUMAN EMBRYO

As explained above, IVF is linked to embryo wastage because it involves the creation of more embryos than are placed in the woman's body. Some of these embryos may be frozen and stored for future use, a procedure that is far from risk-free for the embryo. Some 'spare' embryos may be used in experiments while others may be directly discarded. This raises the question of the moral status of the embryo. It raises the question whether or to what extent the embryo deserves to be respected and protected. In order to answer these questions we must first answer the question:

When does human life begin?

The answer to this question is: at fertilisation. For once a sperm has entered an ovum, a new being has come into existence with intrinsic powers and potentialities quite unlike those of the two gametes. A new human life has begun. That we are talking about a human being cannot be doubted. The new entity is of human origin and alive. Provided its development is not hampered by illness, accident or intentional destruction, it will grow and develop. It will develop into a foetus and, if all goes well, it will be born and grow into a little boy or a little girl, who will grow to become a man or a woman, a mature human being.

The difference between the newly conceived embryo and a human adult is one of maturity only. From the time of fertilisation the development of the human being is gradual and continuous.

Yet there are those who suggest that human life does not start at fertilisation. They say that the embryo cannot be regarded as an individual human being. Often they give this as a reason for supporting embryo research and as a justification for the embryo wastage associated with IVF. There are three arguments often advanced against the view that the early embryo is an individual human being. They may be called the 'twinning argument', the 'placenta argument' and the 'natural wastage' argument.

1) The twinning argument

In the Human Fertilisation and Embryology Act 1990 the fourteenth day after conception, the time of the appearance of the primitive streak, is taken as a decisive cut-off point marking a new life. Thus it is legal to experiment on the embryo or allow it to develop up to the fourteenth day but not beyond.

Why is the fourteenth day, or the development of the primitive streak, considered so special? The answer is that each primitive streak marks out one embryo only and the orientation of the developing embryonic body. The early embryo may cleave and two embryos instead of one may result. Hence it has been argued that until the embryo is observably one it cannot be regarded as an individual being.

However, this argument is faulty. In the first place, the majority of embryos do not twin. Therefore, the majority of embryos are, without a doubt, individual beings, that is, individual human beings, from the time of conception. As for embryos destined to twin, they may encompass two individual lives from the start. They may represent a kind of Siamese twinning, meaning that they share the same body mass. If this is the case, there are two individual presences from the very beginning. There is also the possibility that the early embryo may give rise to a second embryo by a kind of budding. If this is the case, the first embryo, an individual being from the very beginning, remains an individual being. As for the second embryo, it too is an individual being from the time its life begins. But its life starts later than that of the first embryo from whom it sprang. Whatever the explanation of twinning, it casts no doubt on fertilisation as the origin of most - if not all - human beings.

2) The placenta argument

This argument is to the effect that because some of the cells in the early embryo will develop into the placenta and other tissue needed to support the growing foetus, the embryo cannot be regarded as an individual human being. In other words, it is suggested that the foetus may be identified only with those cells that later develop into the 'foetus proper', and that the other cells destined to become placenta and other supportive tissue should be regarded as something separate and different from the foetus. However, this argument too is faulty because the placenta is an integral part of the foetal organism. This is because foetus and placenta develop in unison in a jointly goal-directed manner, and so as a functional unity. That the placental tissue is discarded after birth does not change this. Like the milk-teeth, the placenta is discarded when it is no longer needed.

3) The natural wastage argument

It is often pointed out that the majority of naturally conceived embryos perish. And this is taken to prove that the early embryo is not a human individual. However, this is a poor argument, as is obvious if we remember that in the past a very considerable number of infants and young children perished. So if the same argument had been applied to them, one would have had to draw the conclusion that young children are not human individuals. Few of us would buy that argument.

Even among those who are convinced that human life starts at fertilisation, there are those who argue that the moral status of the embryo is radically different from that of a child or an adult person and that the embryo does not deserve the same respect as more mature human beings. Some of the advocates of this line of argument say that as the unborn child develops senses and faculties such as hearing or the ability to feel pain it is gradually owed more and more respect. Others suggest more or less distinct criteria of humanhood or personhood, such as rationality and a sense of personal identity.

However, most of the characteristics singled out to identify human beings proper, or human persons, are missing not only in the embryo and foetus but also in the infant and even in the young child. But few of us would deny that infants and small children are human beings whose life and integrity ought to be respected and protected.

Moreover, all the different cut-off points and criteria suggested are arbitrary. There is only one moment that marks a morally significant difference: the formation of an embryo - normally at conception, when sperm and ovum combine to form a single entity. Unlike the embryo, neither gamete has an inherent ability to develop into a mature human being. Thus there is a morally significant difference between a gamete and an embryo. Since the development of the embryo is continuous from the time of conception onwards, from this point we are talking about a boy or a girl, about someone like you or me, but one who has only just begun the journey of life. For this reason, the intentional wastage or destruction of embryonic life cannot be justified. The human embryo is our neighbour, a member of the human family. It deserves to be respected and protected from the time of conception.

This rules out IVF involving ovarian stimulation and the creation of numerous embryos, some of whom are wasted, destroyed or exposed to the risks inherent in freezing. It also rules out ICSI and ZIFT inasmuch as they too involve ovarian stimulation to create more embryos than can be implanted.

The Church's teaching on respect for the human embryo

As is observed in *Donum Vitae,* 'no experimental datum can be in itself sufficient to bring us to the recognition of a spiritual soul' (*Donum Vitae,* cpt. 1, para.1). In other words, it is not a question of empirical observation whether or not the early embryo can be described as a human person. Nevertheless, taking into account biological evidence, the Church argues that 'the conclusions of science regarding the human embryo provide a valuable indication for discerning by the use of reason a personal presence at the moment of this first appearance of human life: how could a human individual not be a human person?' (*Ibid.*).

For this reason, the Church insists that from the time of conception the embryo must be shown the utmost respect and should not be treated as a disposable object.

Thus the fruit of human generation, from the first moment of its existence, that is to say from the moment the zygote has formed, demands the unconditional respect that is morally due to the human being in his bodily and spiritual totality. The human being is to be respected and treated as a person from the moment of conception; and therefore from that same moment his rights as a person must be recognised, among which in the first place is the inviolable right of every innocent human being to life (*Donum Vitae,* cpt. 1, para.1).

It should be added that the Church has always taught that it is not for human beings to hamper the process of procreation or to cut short human life at any stage as this may interfere with the fulfilment of divine intentions. Indeed, as is pointed out by John Paul II in his encyclical letter *Evangelium Vitae* of 1995, 'the dignity of this life is linked not only to its beginning, to the fact that it comes from God, but also to its final end, to its destiny of fellowship with God in knowledge and love of Him' (para. 38). In other words, human dignity derives both from the fact that life is a gift from God created in His image and from the fact that God has mapped out the road for the pilgrimage of human life, the destination of which is the Kingdom of God. This is important, for those who find it hard to recognise the image of God in the very first cells at the beginning of life, may nonetheless recognise the human dignity of embryonic human life in the light of its final end.

For if the human embryo is destined to become (and will become, unless it succumbs to an accident or is intentionally destroyed) a mature person in the image of God meant for union with God, then the human embryo must surely already be our neighbour created in the image of God and meant for union with God. And if so, we clearly ought to treat it in a neighbourly way and protect it from harm and exploitation.

Thus the Church rules out abortion as well as embryo wastage and destructive embryo research. Embryo experimentation could only be justified if it were in the interest of the individual embryo exposed to the procedures involved. "If embryos are living, whether viable or not, they must be respected just like any other human person; experimentation on embryos which is not directly therapeutic is illicit" (*Donum Vitae,* cpt. 1, para. 4). In particular, *Donum Vitae* emphasises that "human embryos obtained *in vitro* are human beings and subjects with rights", whose "dignity and right to life must be respected from the first moment of their existence" and that "it is immoral to produce embryos destined to be exploited as disposable 'biological material'" (cpt., 1, para. 5).

The Church likewise condemns embryo freezing and storage because it exposes the embryo to the risk of damage and death:

> The freezing of embryos, even when carried out in order to preserve the life of an embryo - cryopreservation

- constitutes an offence against the respect due to human beings by exposing them to grave risks of death or harm to their physical integrity and depriving them, at least temporarily, of maternal shelter and gestation, thus placing them in a situation in which further offences and manipulation are possible (*Donum Vitae,* cpt. 1. para. 6).

In short, the Church asks us to treat the human embryo as a child, as a member of the human family, as a neighbour in the image of God and as a divine gift. We have a moral responsibility before God for the embryo's welfare. We are not creators. Each new life comes from God, even if human agency is also involved.

In the book of Genesis we read: "And Adam knew Eve his wife; and she conceived and bare Cain, and said, I have gotten a man from the Lord" (*Gn* 4:1). This passage together with Genesis 1:27-28, which states that we are created in the image of God and tells us to rule over the earth, makes it clear that the child born to Eve originated from God as well as from the union of Adam and Eve. It tells us that the child was a gift from God at the same time as it was the result of Adam 'knowing' his wife Eve. That is, the child was the fruit both of the man-woman union and of divine action. Thus Adam and Eve may be jointly described as co-creators with God.

It is also noteworthy that the command to replenish and subdue the earth follows immediately upon the description of the human couple as created in the image of God. This is surely with the implication that it is because the couple are created in the image of God that they have been entrusted with the task and responsibility of subduing the earth. But the call to subdue the earth should not be interpreted as a licence for humans to adopt an instrumentalist attitude towards the rest of creation. The creation of man and woman in the image of God must be understood as conferring a responsibility of stewardship over the rest of creation, including human children until they have reached maturity and are ready to assume their share of the responsibilities involved in human stewardship. Stewardship also entails representation. In other words, when Adam and Eve were told to have dominion over all the living things on earth, they were entrusted with the responsibility of bearing witness to and acting on behalf of God Himself before the rest of creation, not least before their own children.

John Paul II, who has discussed the parent-child relationship at length, says that with biological parenting comes a responsibility to educate the offspring by bearing witness to God (see *Familiaris Consortio,* paras 25, 36-41; *Letter to Families,* para. 16). He also says that this means showing a respectful attitude towards our children as well as bringing them the Gospel news and seeking to live in the spirit of the same Gospel. Speaking of the fourth commandment John Paul II says that the respect owed to parents on the part of children implies that parents should act in such a way that they merit that honour (cf., *Letter to Families,* para 15). But how can they merit respect unless they treat their neighbours created in the image of God in a neighbourly way and so with respect? Not only must children be treated with some minimal respect by their parents and elders, but they must be treated as their equals in human dignity. They must not be treated as human products or property. That children must not be treated as human products or possessions follows from the understanding of the child as a gift from God, in the image of God, received in human co-creation. Viewed as a gift from God entrusted to our care as our neighbour, the child cannot be viewed as an object that we may dispose of as we wish. To treat children as products and possessions is incompatible with that caring and respectful attitude towards the child called for by the parental vocation understood as delegated by God. The child must be protected from the time of conception and he or she ought to be truly begotten, not made, of one being with his or her parents and flesh of their flesh.

THE CHURCH'S TEACHING ON RESPECT FOR THE PARENT-CHILD RELATIONSHIP

The term procreation suggests the creative involvement of God each time a new human life begins. It suggests human co-creation rather than a purely human act. By contrast, the term reproduction suggests that the child is the product of human action alone. It suggests that the child is man-made and solely the result of a human project.

Of course, techniques of artificial reproduction that bypass the union in the flesh encourage the view that the child is a man-made product and a solely human project. The case is different with techniques such as repair of the fallopian tubes, which allow couples to have children by normal intercourse. Not only do techniques of artificial reproduction depersonalise the child, they also depersonalise the very process of generating new life. They turn an act designed by God for personal self-giving into a kind of engineering. When the techniques bypassing sexual intercourse are coupled with gamete donation, the depersonalisation of procreation and the commodification of the child are taken a step further. For then not only has the child been treated as a human product but it has also become the object of a transaction involving an exchange of goods. This is a far cry from being the outcome and sign of parental self-giving.

In *Donum Vitae* all techniques of artificial reproduction that bypass the sexual act and/or involve gamete donation are condemned for reasons that are spelled out below.

Why must the child be the fruit of married love?

We read in *Donum Vitae*:

> Every human being is always to be accepted as a gift and blessing of God. However, from the moral point of view a truly responsible procreation vis-à-vis the unborn child must be the fruit of marriage (cpt 2, para.1).

The reason given for the statement that the child should be the fruit of marriage is that although gamete donation does not strictly speaking involve spousal infidelity it drives a kind of wedge between the couple as well as between them and the child. Gamete donation affects the child's identity as well as the parents' own relationship. This is because, instead of being the fruit of the love of the spouses and thus a living symbol or reflection of their mutual love for one another, the child is the outcome of a type of barter. In other words:

> The procreation of a new person, whereby man and woman collaborate with the power of the Creator, must be the fruit and the sign of the mutual self-giving of the spouses, of their love and their fidelity (cpt 2, para. 1).

In other words, with gamete donation the spousal union is violated, as is the child's meaning as a sign of total mutual self-giving. Thus gamete donation is neither compatible with the exclusiveness of marriage nor with that of the parent-child relationship. It is an insult to both relationships precisely because the child does not spring from the spousal union but comes into being through the intervention or intrusion of a third party, the donor. In his *Letter to Families* of 1994, John Paul II tells us that the child should be seen as completing marriage and as 'the crowning' of married love (para. 9). Similarly, in the Apostolic Exhortation *Familiaris Consortio* of 1981, he says that the child born as the result of the union of the flesh of husband and wife is "a living reflection of their love [...] a permanent sign of conjugal unity and a living and inseparable synthesis of their being a father and a mother" (para. 14). To the mind of John Paul II, when the family is founded in the spousal embrace of mutual self-giving, it becomes, as does the child itself, a sign of God's salvific covenant with man and of the Triune mystery. John Paul II lays great stress on the Trinitarian likeness of the family:

> Human fatherhood and motherhood, while remaining biologically similar to that of other living beings in nature, contain in an essential and unique way a 'likeness' to God, which is the basis of the family as a community of human life, as a community of persons united in love (*communio personarum*).

In the light of the New Testament it is possible to discern how the primordial model of the family is to be sought in God himself, in the Trinitarian mystery of His life (*Letter to Families,* para. 6).

Apart from the deep symbolism he finds in the family and the child, John Paul II also says that, at the personal or relational level, the child springing from the intimate personal and physical communion of the spouses enriches and deepens their relationship at the personal level (*Letter to Families,* para.7). Indeed, John Paul II's symbolic understanding of the child is rooted in his relational or personalistic understanding of the child as a focus of a shared love, who serves - or should serve - to strengthen the bond of love between the spouses. It is as persons in union and communion that spouses as a couple and as parents of a child reflect the Trinitarian union; that is, the communion of Father, Son and Holy Spirit.

Not only does gamete donation violate the spousal union and distort the child's meaning as an expression of that union but it is also an insult to the dignity of the child and a grave injustice that affects its very identity. In *Donum Vitae* we read:

> It is through the secure and recognised relationship to his own parents that the child can discover his own identity and achieve his own proper human development (cpt 2, para 1).

In the case of gamete donation the child is forsaken by one or both of its genetic parents. Gamete donation constitutes a failure on the part of the donor to assume parental responsibility. As *Donum Vitae* emphasises, the child needs to be begotten and reared strictly within marriage for the sake of its healthy psychological development. It needs this in order to feel secure and as a confirmation of its human dignity and worth. But when a donor abdicates his or her parental role as steward, the child is viewed as an object of barter. For to undertake to become a parent in order to alienate one's parental relation to the child is to treat the child not as a person but as a commodity. Even if the donor is paid little or nothing, his or her transaction and that of the recipients involves an 'exchange of goods'. This is to treat the child as a chattel, rather than as our neighbour created in the image of God. It is an insult to the human dignity of the child.

To those who compare gamete donation to adoption it should be pointed out that adoption is, in fact, very different. When a child is adopted the adopting parents accept the care of a child who has been orphaned or given away because its natural mother or parents feel that they cannot take care of it. Unlike a child conceived by means of gamete donation, it would not have been conceived in order to be given away. More probably the child was not planned at all.

It may also be noted that adoption could take place at different stages in the life of the child, even before it is born. In some exceptional cases we might consider embryo adoption justified, though Catholics are divided on the question of whether Church teaching allows this.

For example, women could come forward offering to carry to term embryos who have been abandoned, such as embryos who have been stored up to the legal time limit and whose parents are not contactable for a parental decision about their fate. In the case of abandoned embryos, vicarious parental stewardship might be seen as a kind of rescue operation. This situation is not to be confused with pre-planned embryo donation. With embryo adoption the child is not treated as a commodity but as a person whose life is precious.

In short, the Church teaches that gamete donation is an insult both to the spousal relationship and to the child. This rules out donor insemination as well as IVF, ZIFT and GIFT involving egg or sperm donation, or both.

The Church also rules out other techniques where a child is deliberately conceived and gestated for the benefit of a commissioning couple. It rules out surrogacy, a procedure that has not been mentioned before in this document, since it is not so much a form of fertility treatment as a form of baby trade. Surrogacy may take place in different ways. Often it involves artificial insemination by the male party of the commissioning couple. Alternatively, it may involve embryo transfer to the surrogate mother using the commissioning couple's embryo. If artificial insemination is used and the child carried by the surrogate is her own genetic child, then the surrogate fails to assume her parental responsibility and stewardship when she hands over the child to the commissioning couple. The same is true in the case of embryo transfer inasmuch as the surrogate, as gestational mother, is a biological mother of the child, even if she is not its genetic mother. Surrogacy is an insult both to the surrogate and to the child. It is an insult to the child as our equal and neighbour in the image of God inasmuch as it is treated as an object of barter. It is an insult to the surrogate because she is treated as not much more than a hired prenatal incubator. Whatever the kind of surrogacy arrangement, like all forms of egg, sperm and planned embryo donation, it is an insult to human dignity, since it means treating human beings and body-parts as marketable commodities.

What is wrong with techniques that bypass the sexual act?

In his Apostolic Letter of 1988, *Mulieris Dignitatem,* John Paul II explains that the story of the creation of woman as a 'helper fit for man' shows that human beings are not meant to be alone but are called to interpersonal union and communion with God and neighbour (cf., *Gen* 2:21-25). This, he says, is because the divine life, in whose image man and woman are created, is intrinsically relational. Thus he tells us that marriage was the first way in which human beings were taught to answer the divine call to interpersonal union and communion (*Mulieris Dignitatem,* para. 7). He says that God spoke to us by creating human beings as man and woman and explains that humankind's dual embodiment as man and woman is full of symbolism, revealing truths about our relationship with God and about the inner Trinitarian life of God Himself.

On John Paul II's understanding, the very order of creation has normative implications; it tells us about right and wrong. Our dual nature as man and woman as well as the spousal relationship divinely instituted by God lay down certain rules. The very order of creation lays down rules for the relationship between husband and wife and also for the relationship between parents and children.

However, human beings are prone to create their own rules. Speaking about today's families, John Paul II makes the following observations in *Familiaris Consortio*. Compared with the past, 'there is a more lively awareness of personal freedom and greater attention to the quality of interpersonal relationships in marriage, to promoting the dignity of women, to responsible procreation, the education of children' (para. 6). But while finding much to praise in the present, John Paul II also warns of human hubris, the root of which he finds in the lack of humility reflected in the secular liberal idea of autonomy, which fosters selfishness and represents a denial of the Christian concept of freedom. On John Paul II's understanding, the concept of freedom, perceived in the light of the Gospel, entails a capacity for what is good and right for the human being according to man's divinely ordained nature. In particular, it entails "a capacity for realising the truth of God's plan for marriage and the family" (*ibid.*).

John Paul II tells us that "the family has the mission to guard, reveal and communicate love, and this is the living reflection of and a real sharing in God's love for humanity and the love of Christ the Lord for the Church His bride" (*Familiars Consortio,* para. 17). Thus John Paul II says that "the family which is founded and given life by love is a community of persons" (*Familiars Consortio,* para. 18). By this he means that the family, which springs from the union of husband and wife, forms a truly personal community, a community in which each member is loved and respected as a person, as an equal created in the image of God. This carries the moral implication that the community of the family ought to be the fruit of the full union and communion of the spouses (cf., *Letter to Families,* para. 7). Thus John Paul II says that when, through their mutual self-giving in the body, man and woman beget a child, the child too "becomes a part of the horizon of the 'we' of the spouses, and enters, as a gift from God, their union to make it a community of love, destined for union with God" (*Letter to Families,* para. 11).

In short, John Paul's message is clear: human procreation should be the result of the union in the flesh of man and wife. His message echoes that of *Donum Vitae,* where it is stated that:

In his unique and irrepeatable origin, the child must be respected and recognised as equal in personal dignity to those who give him life. The human person must be accepted in his parents' act of union and love; the generation of a child must therefore be the fruit of that mutual giving which is realised in the conjugal act wherein the spouses co-operate as servants and not as masters in the work of the Creator who is Love.

In reality, the origin of a human person is the result of an act of giving. The one conceived must be the fruit of his parents' love. He cannot be desired or conceived as the product of an intervention of medical or biological techniques; that would be the equivalent to reducing him to an object of scientific technology (*Donum Vitae*, cpt 2, para.4).

In sum, it matters whether the child is co-created in the warmth of the sexual embrace. Manipulative techniques of assisted conception encourage the view that procreation is a solely human project and the child a product, inherent in which view is a disrespectful attitude towards the child. Such techniques depersonalise the act of begetting. The intervention of a third party in this very act, a party more actively involved in the conception of the child than the spouses themselves, also reduces the father and the mother to raw material for a process of making. The father and the mother become objects of manipulation rather than procreators. They, like the child-to-be, fall under the domination of technology. As explained in *Donum Vitae:* "It sometimes happens that a medical procedure technologically replaces the conjugal act in order to obtain a procreation which is neither its result nor its fruit. In this case the medical act is not, as it should be, at the service of conjugal union but rather appropriates to itself the procreative function and thus contradicts the dignity and inalienable rights of the spouses and of the child to be born" (cpt 2, para. 7).

In the light of these reflections, let us consider AIH as well as GIFT and IVF not involving gamete donation.

AIH

While the child conceived by AIH may be conceived within marriage, nevertheless the technique violates the requirement that the child should be the fruit of parental union in the flesh. The technique is manipulative and bypasses the union in the flesh of husband and wife. This, as argued above, effectively means treating the child as a product and distorting the child's symbolic meaning. It makes the child a product of human technology, rather than a living proof of spousal love and its expression of intimate self-giving in the human embrace. Thus *Donum Vitae* explains that AIH is wrong because the conception of the child is not the result of "the mutual gift, which, according to the words of the Scripture, brings about union 'in one flesh'". (*Donum Vitae*, cpt. 2, para.6). To put it differently, the child is not the crowning of spousal love in the image of Trinitarian love.

Furthermore, that child does not spring from the human embrace but is the product of a technological intervention on the part of a third party. This depersonalises not only the child but also the parents and the very act of conception. Technology has taken over. When the parents subject themselves in this way to the dominion of technology, the act of procreation is no longer strictly speaking theirs. Their personal involvement is not active but passive. It is precisely for this reason that, unlike the child co-created in the spousal union in the flesh, the child resulting from technology cannot be seen as the crowning and living reflection of spousal love in all its intimacy, itself a reflection of the inner life of the One and Triune God.

GIFT involving no gamete donation is similar to AIH, and the Church therefore rules it out for much the same reasons as it rules out AIH.

IVF

IVF is open to the same objection as AIH, namely that the spousal act of procreation has been usurped by technology, which depersonalises the spouses and the child as well as the act of procreation. Indeed, IVF is an even more manipulative and technological procedure than AIH, in that multiple embryos are conceived outside the

mother's body. Here the child really is reduced to a
product rather than received as a gift and sign of the
fullness of spousal love.

IVF is disrespectful of embryonic human life and for this
reason particularly is morally unacceptable. As shown
above, every IVF embryo is vulnerable to harmful
exploitation. The very fact that the embryo - our young
neighbour created in the image of God - is in the petri-dish
exposes it to human caprice and manipulation. IVF is a
threat to its life and an insult to its human dignity. We have
seen that normally many embryos are created at one time,
while only one or two are chosen for implantation. The
others are frozen, destroyed or experimented on, all of which
means wanton loss of human life. Some people object to this
argument by pointing out that even with natural conception
and pregnancy many embryos are lost. But, as we have seen,
this objection is irrelevant. We have no responsibility for
what is not under our control, and therefore no responsibility
for embryonic losses due to nature. But we do have a
responsibility for our own actions. We do have a
responsibility for how we treat human embryonic life. If our
manipulations expose the human embryo to injury and
death, we are morally answerable for this.

In sum, IVF violates the child's symbolic meaning as
an expression of spousal union in the fullness of the flesh
and it is also an expression of an instrumental attitude
towards the child-to-be. It brings the embryo into being

like an artefact - a disposable artefact. It is the intentional producing of embryos in a manner that leaves them open to deliberate harm and injury. When IVF is used in conjunction with gamete or embryo donation, the child is doubly wronged at the same time as the exclusiveness of the spousal union is violated.

CONCLUSION

Having examined the field of reproductive technology, we have made a distinction between, on the one hand, procedures that restore reproductive function or otherwise assist couples to have children by normal intercourse, and on the other, procedures that replace normal intercourse by technology and which may even make use of donor gametes or donor embryos in order to establish a pregnancy. Only in the case of the former kind of procedure is the child received not as a product but as a gift: a gift that reflects and is a sign of total and exclusive spousal self-giving.

Looking at the second kind of procedure we find, by contrast, a slippery slope that has brought us ever closer towards the ultimate commodification of the child as well as the ultimate depersonalisation of procreation. Increasingly, what God joined together at the beginning, namely sexual intercourse and procreation, are being separated by modern technology. For with modern reproductive technology it is possible to have babies without having sex. It is possible to have babies using donated gametes or embryos. It is possible to create embryos outside the maternal body. It is possible to separate gestational motherhood from genetic motherhood. Our final feat, which some claim has already been achieved, is the separation of procreation of new human life from fertilisation - that is, human cloning. Cloning involves neither the coupling of spouses nor the coupling of gametes.

When technological manipulation takes control over reproduction, men, women and children are depersonalised. Indeed, a whole new terminology has been developed that bears witness to depersonalisation and commodification in the area of assisted conception. Terms such as 'products of conception' for children, 'harvesting' for egg retrieval and 'surrogate uteruses' or 'reproduction vehicles' for women as well as 'collection of semen' speak for themselves. Such terms dehumanise men, women and children. Women are fragmented into ovaries, wombs and eggs, which may be part exchanged, rented or donated to produce the commodity child. The man is used as little more than a stud. The child is treated as an object both of production and of barter; and as such it is subjected to quality control, selection and storage. The child put together in the laboratory is not given that unconditional welcome that every child deserves. It is not treated as a gift and new member of the family to be unconditionally accepted, cherished and protected.

However, while the child should be cherished as a gift and a new member of the family, and while it has been described as the crowning of the spousal relationship and a reflection of spousal love, it should not for that reason be concluded that the union of spouses who are not capable of having children does not have its own value.

Childlessness as well as parenthood may be seen as a vocation. Not only may the childless state have its own kind of fruitfulness by way of creative work and taking care of others, it may also have its own unitive powers bringing the spouses ever closer and making their union an ever truer reflection of Trinitarian love and of the love of Christ our Lord for the Church (cf., *Eph* 5:21-33).

Couples should not bring themselves to think that they 'must' have a child. However, they may, of course, take whatever steps are reasonable to conceive. If they try to conceive by seeking medical assistance, they ought carefully to reflect on the kind of medical advice and help they seek. This is the message of this booklet and it is hoped that the booklet will help those who read it to see that it matters what kind of assistance couples choose. It matters for the spousal relationship and it matters for the parents' relationship with the prospective child.

If couples remain childless, not only might they consider adoption, but they might also consider how to live fruitful lives without children. Without children they will have more time for God and neighbour as well as for one another. They will have more time for nourishing friendships as well as for other ways of being spiritually fruitful.

While children are blessings and gifts from God, they are not to be had at any cost. They deserve to enter the world not as manufactured goods but as our equals conceived in the warmth of a loving embrace.

FURTHER READING

These documents are all available from CTS.

Sacred Congregation for the Doctrine of the Faith, *Declaration on Procured Abortion,* 1974.

John Paul II, *Familiaris Consortio,* 1981. (S 357)

Congregation for the Doctrine of the Faith, *Donum Vitae,* 1987 (published by the CTS as The Gift of Life).

John Paul II, Apostolic Letter *Mulieris Dignitatem* (The Dignity of Women), 1988. (Do 584)

John Paul II, *Letter to Families,* 1994. (S 434)

John Paul II, Encyclical Letter *Evangelium Vitae* (The Gospel of Life), 1995. (Do 633)

CONTACTS

Linacre Centre for Healthcare Ethics, tel: (020) 7806 4088;
e-mail: *admin@linacre.org* website: *www.linacre.org*
Provides moral advice on fertility tests and treatments.

Life Fertility Programme, tel: 0151 228 0353;
e-mail: *info@lifefertility.co.uk* website: *www.lifefertility.co.uk*

Other centres offering Naprotechnology are listed at
www.naprotechnology.com

GLOSSARY

Abortifacient: something (e.g. a drug) that has the effect of producing an abortion

Abortion: the killing of an unborn child

Amniotic fluid: fluid surrounding the foetus within the amniotic sac in the uterus (womb)

Amniotic sac: sac of fluid surrounding the unborn child during pregnancy

AID: artificial insemination by husband

DI: artificial insemination with donor semen

Anaesthesia: procedure or medication that produces a loss of sensation

Artificial insemination: injection of semen into a woman's vagina

Cervical mucus: mucus secreted by the cervix, or neck of the womb

Conception: the union of the ovum (egg) and sperm (also called fertilisation)

Conceptus: unborn child

Ectopic pregnancy: a medical condition in which the embryo starts growing outside the uterus (womb), usually in the fallopian tube

Embryo: unborn child from the time of fertilisation to some two months later

Embryo biopsy: removal of one or more cells from the embryo for examination (also called pre-implantation diagnosis)

Embryogenesis: embryo development

Endocrine glands: hormone-secreting glands

Endometriosis: a condition involving misplaced endometrial tissue (lining of the womb) in the pelvic area

Endometrium: lining of the uterus (womb)

Extra-corporeal fertilisation: fertilisation outside the body

Foetus: unborn child from the end of the second month until birth

Fertilisation: the union of ovum (egg) and sperm (also called conception)

Fibroids: benign tumours in the uterus (womb)

Follicle: see ovarian follicle

Gamete: sperm or ovum

Gestation: the period of the development of the unborn child in the uterus (womb)

GIFT: gamete intra-fallopian transfer, a surgical procedure involving the transfer of ova (eggs) and sperm to the fallopian tube

Gynaecology: the branch of medicine concerned with disorders of the female reproductive system

Hormone: a chemical substance secreted into the blood by the endocrine glands in order to control bodily processes or stimulate other glands

Immune system: the body's defence system against invading organisms such as bacteria and viruses

***In vitro* fertilisation (IVF):** the creation of an embryo outside the maternal body

Laparoscope: a long narrow telescope, which can be passed through the abdominal wall to inspect internal organs

Laparoscopy: visualisation of internal organs by means of a laparoscope

Menopause: the permanent cessation of menstrual periods

Menstrual cycle: the regular monthly changes in the woman's body which control ovulation and menstruation

Menstruation: the woman's monthly loss of blood

Multiple pregnancy: a pregnancy with more than one child

Non-therapeutic: non-healing

Non-therapeutic research: research that is not aimed at benefiting the research subject

Obstetrics: the branch of medicine concerned with the pregnant woman and her unborn child

Oestrogen: a major female hormone

Ovarian follicle: a minute sac within the ovary from which the ovum (egg) is released

Ovarian stimulation: hormone treatment to induce ovulation, sometimes with a view to producing several ripe ova (eggs) in one cycle

Ovary: female reproductive organ producing the ova (eggs). The woman has two ovaries: one on each side of the uterus

Ovum (plural ova): female reproductive cell or egg, which may be fertilised to create an embryo

Pelvic inflammatory disease: infection of the ovaries and fallopian tubes

Pelvis: the body basin containing the pelvic organs, e.g. the reproductive organs and the bladder

Placenta: the organ (of foetal origin) in the uterus (womb) from which the foetus gets its nourishment from the maternal blood via the umbilical cord

Post-coital: after intercourse

Premature birth: birth before the 37th week of pregnancy

Prenatal diagnosis: diagnosis of a medical condition in the foetus

Pre-implantation diagnosis: diagnosis of a medical condition in the embryo created by IVF. (See embryo biopsy.)

Primary infertility: infertility in a couple - or a woman - with no previous child

Primitive streak: longitudinal axis in the developing embryo, which appears around the 14th day after fertilisation

Procured abortion: deliberate abortion

Progesterone: a major female hormone

Secondary infertility: infertility in a couple - or a woman - with a previous child

Semen: fluid (normally containing millions of sperms) emitted from a man's penis at orgasm

Seminal fluid: see semen

Sperm: the male reproductive cell, which may fertilise the ovum (egg) to produce an embryo

Subfertility: impaired fertility

Super-ovulation: hormone stimulation to encourage production of a number of ova (eggs) in the same menstrual cycle

Testis (plural testes): male reproductive organ that produces sperm

Testosterone: the main male sex hormone

Therapeutic: healing

Therapeutic research: research aimed at benefiting the subject

Ultrasound scan: a non-invasive test involving visualisation of the foetus on a screen

Zygote: the single-cell embryo

Informative Catholic Reading

We hope that you have enjoyed reading this booklet.

If you would like to find out more about CTS booklets - we'll send you our free information pack and catalogue.

Please send us your details:

Name ....

Address ....

....

....

Postcode ....

Telephone..

Email ....

Send to: CTS, 40-46 Harleyford Road,
            Vauxhall, London
            SE11 5AY

Tel: 020 7640 0042
Fax: 020 7640 0046
Email: info@cts-online.org.uk

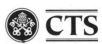